Just Barbell

Power Through

Men & Woman

Break through that wall, build a strong foundation
and core, build muscle and strength. Look and feel
fantastic. There is no other routine like this.

Routine and Daily Logbook

Just Barbell

Designed and created – Stephen John Peel

Cover – Stephen John Peel

© 2020StephenJohnPeel

info@stephenpeel.co.uk

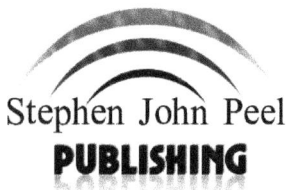

ISBN: 978-0-244-28324-7

Introduction

At the time of writing this, I'm 57 years old, and I have been lifting weights for most of my life. I own a vitamin and supplement company and know a thing or two about fitness and nutrition. Just a little about me, and that's enough.

- This routine is for you if you're just starting and want to build a robust and stable frame that will set you up for the rest of your life

- You're starting in strength training and dreaming of becoming a bodybuilder or Strongman or Strongwoman

- You've been training for years, and you've hit a wall

For the next six months, you'll use nothing but an Olympic barbell in the gym, with weights attached of course. To warm-up, you'll do 15 minutes of cardio, like on a treadmill or exercise bike. Better still, walk or cycle to the gym if it's 15 minutes to half an hour away.

You'll use an Olympic barbell because it's generally thicker than some other barbells, and it will help to strengthen your grip and forearm strength. It will sit much more comfortably on your shoulders when doing squats, and it weighs 20 kilograms or 44 pounds.

If you're expecting pages and pages, with me babbling on with detailed and longwinded instructions, then look for another book. You don't need me to explain how to complete every exercise.

Other than watching instructional YouTube videos for each exercise, the best thing you can do is book an hour or two with an instructor at your local gym. The instructor will go over each of the exercises I've included here so that you'll know how to perform them safely.

When it comes to nutrition, you don't need me to tell you how to eat either. It's common sense. You already know what's right and wrong. But if you're unsure, let me explain.

Steak and salad = good, a bucket of fried chicken = bad.

Not clear enough? Okay, I'll try again.

Kippers, toast, or boiled eggs for breakfast with orange juice and black coffee = good. Pancakes or sugar-coated cereal with a milkshake and coffee with milk and sugar = bad. How simple is that?

Your body won't thank you for a doughnut, but it will reward you for a lean chicken breast. I've mentioned mainly meats there, but you vegans and veggies will be able to work out what's best for you, as you no doubt already do.

I suggest you take an excellent multivitamin and mineral tablet each day with your healthy diet. Other than that, you're good to go.

Oh, and make sure you're physically capable of carrying out the exercises without injury. If you have health issues, see your doctor for advice before doing these exercises. Get a qualified gym instructor to advise. Disclaimer complete.

Let's get started

You'll spend at least one-hour training each training day. Ideally, you'll train five or six days per week, but if you can only manage three days, so be it. This routine will still work amazingly.

Don't set days; just say you're going to train three, five or six days a week or even seven. That way, if ever you want a day off, you can take any day of the week.

Workouts

Let me say this before you start working out. Don't go playing on machines or cables during your workout. If you have a few minutes to kill at the end of the session, sure, play around on the other equipment, but don't stress your muscles out on them, you're going to need them.

For the whole of your one-hour workout, you'll do only one or two exercises. It might be bench-pressing or squats, for example, or it could be a combination of a flat bench and inclined bench.

You'll look at the clock, your watch or phone, and every time the big hand reaches a five-minute increment; it will then be time to start another set. So if one set of ten reps takes you one minute to complete, you'll have four minutes rest before then next. Don't rush.

You could get as many as 12 sets in your hour, but ten will be fine. These exercises will take it out of you. You might think an hour isn't long enough, or that you'll not feel you've done sufficiently by doing one exercise, but trust me, you'll have done plenty, and you'll feel it. Drink plenty of water before and during each workout. Your muscles will need it.

After four weeks on this routine, stop for one week. In that week, keep going to the gym, but enjoy playing around on all the other machines and contraptions. You'll have no doubt been staring at them and longing, so reward yourself and spend a week on them, then get back to this routine for the next four weeks. You'll be doing this for a whole six months.

Now don't get me wrong, there is nothing at all wrong with cables, machines or dumbbells, they're all excellent. But this routine is designed to build a strong solid foundation and core for beginners, or break through a wall and shake things up a bit for the more experienced.

It's a routine designed for everyone interested in healthy bones and joints, powerful muscles, ligaments and tendons. It will set you up for life. If you like the routine, you can benefit from six months on and six months of other training, continually, but see how you go.

Your Details

	Start	Finish
Name		
Contact		
Height		
Weight		
Body Measurements		
Neck		
Shoulders		
Chest		
Biceps and Triceps		
Forearms		
Waist		
Hips		
Butt		
Thighs		
Calves		

Workout One – Squats

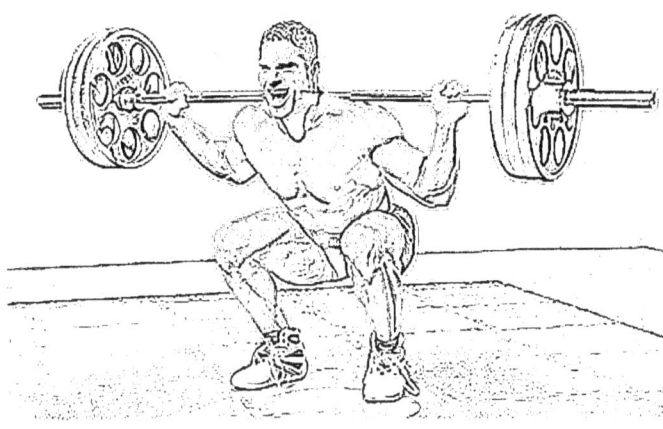

This exercise, for a whole hour, will have you feeling great, if not a little exhausted, and maybe even sore.

Your muscles need to mend after each workout, but keeping moving is essential. There'll be no resting up for days on end, and you'll go straight into the next exercise in the next session.

Your first set will be 15 reps with just the bar. Some of you will find that the bar is heavy enough, and that's okay. Stick to the just the bar for as many reps as you can up to 15, and if you don't think you'll manage any extra weight, that's fine. Don't rush it. Rushing will lead to injury.

For those that find the bar easy, load it up with 5 or 10 kg per side and go for ten reps on your second set. Your first set must remain 15 reps. If you can't make ten reps on the second, that's okay, take some weight off. Continue doing set after set at five minutes intervals with as much on your shoulders as you can manage safely for ten reps.

For those muscle-bound strongmen and women, keep adding a little weight for each set until you can't get ten reps, then take some weights off and get that ten reps. Don't try to do low reps with massive loads. That will do you no good at all and could result in injury. Stick to ten for this routine.

Make sure you also use clips on the barbell to stop the weights sliding off, and always use a squat cage, or have support bars set lower than your squat, just in case you fall or your legs give up on you. Better safe than sorry. Also, stay away from the Smith Machine; it isn't a loose barbell.

These exercises take a lot out of you; they're hard work, which is why most people stay clear of some of them.

Squat Benefits

The squat is an incredible exercise. It's not only a leg exercise, but it will also strengthen your core, your upper and lower back, your shoulders. Quadriceps hamstrings and calves will get a great workout, but so will the rest of your body.

It might take some time to get used to sitting the bar across your shoulders behind your head, but you're in no rush, you'll find the sweet spot. If it's too painful, most gyms have a foam pad that fits around the bar. If they don't have one, get your own. However, I believe that you're better off not using paddy. You'll soon adapt.

Eight of the many benefits

1. Flexibility and focus

Getting up from a chair, climbing stairs, picking up objects, will all become more manageable, and you'll focus as you do those things. Being more flexible and muscular means less chance of injury.

2. Great looking legs

Enough said

3. Posture

Your core will strengthen, and you'll become more upright. You'll think before you move. Your posture depends on the muscles in the front and rear of your body. Sturdy, well-worked muscles, equals better posture.

4. Strong bones, less injury

Load bearing exercises like squatting, thicken and strengthen your bones. But not to the point that someone else will notice, so don't be concerned that someone will see your bones from the outside. Strong bones mean less injury.

5. Heart health

It takes a lot of effort to squat, and your cardiac muscles will strengthen as a result. Your lung capacity will also improve.

6. Increased jumping height

Not that you need to jump, but if you have to, or want to, squatting helps. What your new jumping ability will show is how well developed your legs and core muscles have become.

7. Confidence boosting

When you feel healthy, you feel more confident. You feel physically powerful and look great.

8. Burn fat

The more muscle you have, the more calories you burn, and squats will help build muscle throughout your body like no other exercise.

Workout Two – Standing Shoulder Press

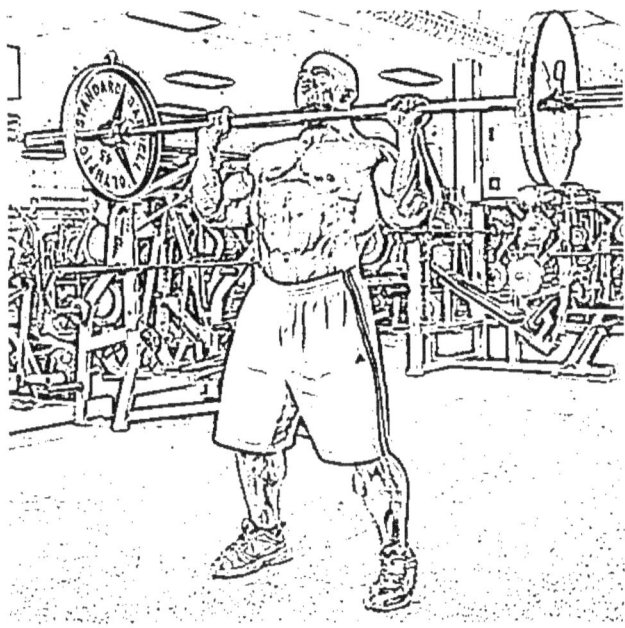

Stack the barbell at the same height in the squat rack as you did for squats. Get yourself under it with your palms facing away from you and your hands at shoulder-width apart. With a slightly curved back, push the barbell up into the air.

You'll find that your head goes back as you try to move the bar as you would in a bench press, but as the bar goes past your forehead, bring your head forward and in line with your body. That's pretty much it, but videos and your gym instructor will put you right and posture.

Upper body strength is evident in the overhead barbell press. This exercise will not only increase the size of your shoulder muscles, but it will also strengthen your core, legs, and most other parts of your body.

Like most of the other compound movements you'll be doing in this routine, the standing overhead barbell press is one of the best. This press is not an easy movement to master. It requires core strength, concentration and body awareness. But you're in no rush, you've got a year to get it right, so take it easy and think before you move.

Four of the many benefits

1. Great shoulders

The barbell shoulder press is the best shoulder exercise. It will help to build broad shoulders and your upper chest. The anterior and medial deltoids are the prime movers, but the traps and rear deltoids also join the party.

2. A rock-solid core

Pushing the weight up in the air pushes you firmly to the ground, and it's up to your core to protect your spine and joints. Stomach muscles and lower back muscles will strengthen and develop.

3. Great traps

This exercise helps develop your traps, but not to the point that they will look overly thick.

4. Complete body workout

Like most of these exercises, you're likely going to need to keep a towel nearby to soak up the sweat. The shoulder press has the whole body working, and you're going to feel it.

Workout Three – Bent Over Rows

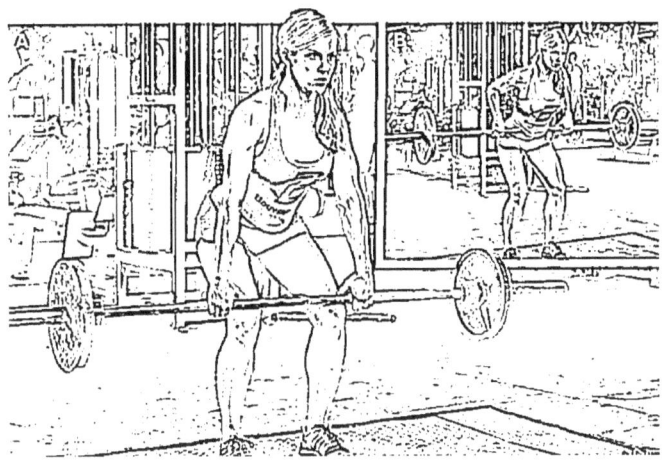

I've gone for bent-over rows and not the deadlift. The squat covers the legs, and we need something that will encourage **latissimus dorsi**, rear delt and trap muscle development. We also have six workouts in this routine, so we have a lot to cover. I don't want you to dread working out with two massive exercises like the squat and the deadlift.

Don't get me wrong. The bent-over barbell row is a tough exercise, and you'll be exhausted after an hour.

Four of the many benefits

1. Complete body workout

Your whole body is once again needed to keep you stable. Leaning over with heavyweight is no easy task. Your legs lower back and core will be in play, not just your upper back muscles. Your arms will ache, and your overhand grip will be hard going. Do not use wrist straps. I want you to develop your wrist and forearm strength and grip.

2. Burn calories

All these exercises burn calories, but you'll no doubt feel the calories vanishing with bent-over rows. The back muscles are enormous, and you'll keep burning calories long after the exercise is complete.

3. Build muscle mass

The back gets neglected like cutting a fringe but leaving a mullet. You rarely see it unless you use two mirrors. It's a shame because a healthy back is attractive and more beautiful than a great looking front to many.

4. Balanced physique

A strong back is essential for balancing your physique. All front and no back would not only look silly, but it would also be unhealthy. When doing barbell rows, you'll find that you can pull a similar weight to what you can push when bench pressing. This balance is needed.

Workout Four – Bench Press

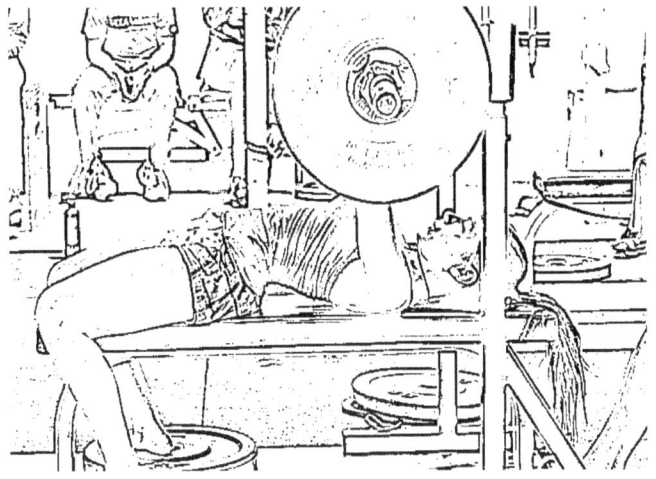

Bent over rows involves pulling, but for bench press, you're going to lie on a flat bench and push the weight away from you.

The bench press is one of the most popular exercises in the gym, especially with the men. So much so, that you'll find it hard to get on a bench on a Monday.

Why is it so popular? Well, you get to lay down for a start. The chest is also a part of the body that receives the most attention. A big chest, or at least one that holds itself up, is to be admired. I don't mean stared at okay.

The bench press is an exercise you can mix up a bit. If you want, use the first half-hour on a flat bench, and the other half-hour on an inclined bench. You'll find that your upper chest and shoulders take over on the incline, and you won't be able to press as much weight as you do on a flat bench.

If the usual bench press stations are in use, go to the squat racks or other frames and see if you can safely drag a bench there and use those.

If you are entirely out of luck finding a station to do any part of your routine, go to the next exercise and back to the one you missed the following day. For example, the next activity after bench press is bicep curls. So you'll do bicep curls, with reverse curls, then bench press the next workout day. But the following week, you'll get the exercises back in line.

It might be harder to work specific muscles out of the order I've given here, but if there's no other option, there's no other option. Don't choose dumbbell or cables or machines to replace the barbell. There's nothing wrong with them, but they're not for this routine.

All these exercises will strengthen and build your core muscles, so no need for situps in this routine.

Five of the many benefits

1. Upper body strength

The main benefit of the bench press is that it will increase upper body strength. The bench press utilizes many different muscles, and the more weight you lift, the more the upper body muscles will be in use.

2. A great chest

Most people aren't thinking of upper body strength when pressing, they're thinking of a big or firm chest, and the bench press will deliver.

3. Triceps are in play

Your triceps will come into play, and they'll need to develop in strength and size as the weight your pushing increases.

4. Burn calories

You may be on a bench, but your focus will be on driving your feet firmly into the floor. Your back will arch slightly so that your upper back is pressed firmly into the bench, and your whole upper body needs to push the weight up into the air. It takes a lot of effort. All these exercises do, and you'll burn a lot of calories.

5. Shoulder workout

If you're switching between flat and declined bench, you'll find your shoulders will take a beating. On a flat, your whole chest gets a workout, but on an incline, chest muscles a little higher up are getting worked, and so are your shoulders. The standing press you've done targets the top part of your chest, but more of your shoulders.

Workout Five – Standing Bicep Curls

The barbell curl is the ultimate bicep exercise. The Olympic bar is heavy. Curling a 20 kg or 44-pound bar without swinging it up will take some doing for those of you just starting, or for those not as developed or as naturally strong in the bicep department as others.

If you can't get at least eight reps out of using the Olympic bar on its own, stop using the bar and go for a smaller bar that has weights already attached. Most gyms have a rack with smaller bars like that. There are also smaller bars that look like the Olympic bar that you can add weights.

Do not use an EZ style bent bar. You must get used to holding a straight bar for every exercise. It will strengthen your wrists, grip and forearms and set you up for the future.

If you can't work with the Olympic bar, stick to the smaller fixed weighted straight bars for a while. It won't be long before you're onto the Olympic bar unweighted. It could be a few months away, but you'll get there.

If you're okay with the Olympic bar, start your workout the same as you do with the other exercises, with 15 reps, then ten reps for every additional set.

The weight you'll need to add at each set will be small—2.5 kg per side. The next will be 5 kg per side, and so on until you've reached your maximum weight for ten reps. Continue the remaining sets at your maximum weight.

After half an hour of curls with your palms facing up, unload the bar and face your palms down using an overhand grip.

For the next half hour, you'll be doing reverse curls to target the outer heads of your biceps and upper forearms. Those of you not on the Olympic bar, do the same with the lighter fixed weight bars until you can work up to the Olympic bar.

Five of the many benefits

1. Bigger biceps

Say no more

2. Everyday lifting

All these exercises will help you in everyday life, from lifting to climbing stairs and so on.

3. Assists other exercises

Muscular biceps are needed to pull the weight in barbell rows, pick up weights and load the bars for all the other exercises in the routine. Without muscular biceps, many of these exercises would be much harder to complete.

4. Full body workout

When it comes to standing barbell curls, the whole of your body is needed to maintain a strict stance while raising the weight. Your legs, core, upper body and back, all engage. Don't be tempted to swing the weight up, it will leave the rest of your body out, and your gains will be limited.

5. Forearm strength

Perfect form is essential for all of the exercises, and slow, deliberate movements will build the body you want, much faster than quick, jerky lifts and presses. Slow and steady on the curl will help develop and strengthen your forearms.

Workout Six – Close Grip Lying Triceps Extensions

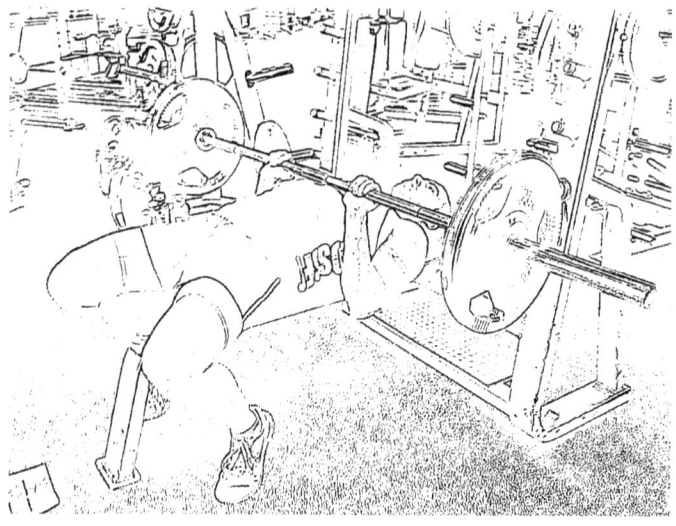

Back on the bench; set yourself up as you do with a bench press. This time, you'll bring your hands in on the bar to shoulder width, or even a tiny little bit closer. With the bench press, your hands will usually be a little bit wider than shoulder-width. But you have to set yourself up the most comfortable way you can, as with any exercise.

Next, you'll lower the Olympic bar to just under your chest, keeping your elbows close to your body. They don't need to touch your body, only slightly off, or whatever feels comfortable. Your grip will be the same as with the bench press, with your palms facing away from you. Your gym instructor will be able to help set you up correctly.

Sets and reps are the same as every other exercise—fifteen reps with just the bar to start, followed by ten reps per set. After half an hour, you'll switch to skull crushers.

You don't have to leave the bench for skull crushers, but you will have to reduce the weight to just the bar to start your 15 reps. To perform this exercise, move your hands along the bar until they're at shoulder width, just like with lying triceps extensions. Then lower the bar to behind the top of your head, keeping your elbows close to your body, then press back up.

The skull crusher, combined with the close grip bench press, will do wonders for your triceps, but keep the weight light on crushers and don't try to overdo it. They're called skull crushers for a reason. If you're not yet strong enough to do this with the Olympic bar, use a smaller weighted bar from the rack until you're strong enough to handle the Olympic.

Three of the many benefits

1. Increase injury resistance

When done safely and correctly, the crushers will ease the risk of injury to the elbow joint and improve extension ability.

2. Build and strengthen

Close grip bench press and skull crushers will build and strengthen all three heads of the triceps, which will enable you to lift more weight in other exercises.

3. Upper chest development

Close grip bench will not only build triceps, but it will add size to your upper chest.

Let's get started

Remember, these exercises need to be completed in order, one workout after the other. Don't mix them up yourself, unless the benches or other equipment are unavailable when you arrive in the gym. If that's the case, do the next exercise and get back on track as soon as you can.

The first set is always 15 reps. The others are ten. If you can't do ten, lower the weight. If you're exhausted towards the end of the workout, and you can only manage a few reps of what you were doing ten of, lower the weight and get ten.

Start new sets as the big hand hits the 5-minute points on the clock, watch, or any other timepiece you might have. Eat well and healthy, and take the right multivitamin and mineral tablet daily.

Watch videos and get instruction from a professional gym instructor on how to perform each of the exercises safely and correctly. Don't let the instructor talk you into an EZ bar, cables, dumbbells or machines, or any other activities for that matter. Those exercises will be useful, but that's not what this routine is all about.

Here are 26 workout pages for you to record the six months you'll be doing this routine. After six months, it's up to you what you do. Try your best to stick to this routine, and it will set you up for the rest of your life, from general fitness to possibly becoming the next world strongest man or woman.

If you only manage three workouts in a week – for example, do the other three the following week. Don't start again from the beginning. One after the other until you've completed all six, then start again. It might seem strange filling out the weeks in different orders, depending on how your workouts run, but you'll get used to it.

Week - Example	Day Date	Max Inc Bar	Number of Sets	How I Feel
Squat	Mon	60 lb	12	Sore
	1 Jan			

Standing Press	Tues	44 lb	10	Tired
	2 Jan			

Bent Over Rows	Thurs	70 lb	10	Great
	4 Jan			

Bench Press	Sat	70 lb	5	Sore
Inclined Press	6 Jan	50 lb	5	Sore

Standing Bicep Curl	Missed			
Reverse Curl				

Close Grip Bench	Missed			
Skull Crushers				

Notes:

_____

_____

_____

_____

_____

_____

_____

Week - Example	Day Date	Max Inc Bar	Number of Sets	How I Feel
Squat	Wed 10 Jan	40 kg	10	Great

Standing Press	Thurs 11 Jan	20 kg	11	Sore

Bent Over Rows	Friday 12 Jan	50 kg	12	Great

Bench Press Inclined Press	Missed			

Next exercise

Standing Bicep Curl Reverse Curl	Mon 8 Jan	40 kg 20 kg	5 5	Great

Close Grip Bench Skull Crushers	Tue 9 Jan	40 kg 20 kg	5 5	Sore

Notes:

_____

_____

_____

_____

_____

_____

_____

Explaination of examples, of those not quite sure

The first example week, you missed two workout sessions.

You then started the following week with the workouts you missed the previous week.

You missed the standing bicep and reverse curls in example week one, so you started the example week one with the standing bicep and reverse curls. Date Mon 8 Jan.

You then followed the Mon 8 Jan with Tues 9 Jan, before going to the top of that workout page to continue with Squats on Wed 10 Jan.

In the second example week, you missed bench and inclined presses, so you'll start the following week with that exercise.

I'm sure that's clear. If not, have someone you know to explain it. I've also used lbs in the first example, and kg in the second. For those that use one or the other.

The notes section at the bottom of each workout page is for you to add anything extra about your workout, as sort of journal.

For example, you might have arrived late at night, and it was great because there was nobody there.

Or you forgot to take your water bottle. Or for anything at all.

Look out for my other journal and logbook. It is a simple set up like this, but you'll be able to enter all your exercises. It will be useful for when you've finished your six months with this routine, or for the weeks you use the machines, cables and dumbbells.

Week - 1	Day Date	Max Inc Bar	Number of Sets	How I Feel
Squat				

	Day Date	Max Inc Bar	Number of Sets	How I Feel
Standing Press				

Bent Over Rows				

Bench Press				
Inclined Press				

Standing Bicep Curl				
Reverse Curl				

Close Grip Bench				
Skull Crushers				

Notes:

_____

_____

_____

_____

_____

_____

_____

Week - 2	Day Date	Max Inc Bar	Number of Sets	How I Feel
Squat				

Standing Press				

Bent Over Rows				

Bench Press				
Inclined Press				

Standing Bicep Curl				
Reverse Curl				

Close Grip Bench				
Skull Crushers				

Notes:

_____

_____

_____

_____

_____

_____

_____

Week - 3	Day Date	Max Inc Bar	Number of Sets	How I Feel
Squat				

Standing Press				

Bent Over Rows				

Bench Press				
Inclined Press				

Standing Bicep Curl				
Reverse Curl				

Close Grip Bench				
Skull Crushers				

Notes:

_____

_____

_____

_____

_____

_____

_____

Week - 4	Day Date	Max Inc Bar	Number of Sets	How I Feel
Squat				
Standing Press				
Bent Over Rows				
Bench Press				
Inclined Press				
Standing Bicep Curl				
Reverse Curl				
Close Grip Bench				
Skull Crushers				

Notes:

_____

_____

_____

_____

_____

_____

_____

Week - 5	Day Date	Max Inc Bar	Number of Sets	How I Feel
Squat				

Standing Press				

Bent Over Rows				

Bench Press				
Inclined Press				

Standing Bicep Curl				
Reverse Curl				

Close Grip Bench				
Skull Crushers				

Notes:

_____

_____

_____

_____

_____

_____

_____

Week - 6	Day Date	Max Inc Bar	Number of Sets	How I Feel
Squat				

Standing Press				

Bent Over Rows				

Bench Press				
Inclined Press				

Standing Bicep Curl				
Reverse Curl				

Close Grip Bench				
Skull Crushers				

Notes:

_____
_____
_____
_____
_____
_____
_____

Week - 7	Day Date	Max Inc Bar	Number of Sets	How I Feel
Squat				

	Day Date	Max Inc Bar	Number of Sets	How I Feel
Standing Press				

	Day Date	Max Inc Bar	Number of Sets	How I Feel
Bent Over Rows				

	Day Date	Max Inc Bar	Number of Sets	How I Feel
Bench Press				
Inclined Press				

	Day Date	Max Inc Bar	Number of Sets	How I Feel
Standing Bicep Curl				
Reverse Curl				

	Day Date	Max Inc Bar	Number of Sets	How I Feel
Close Grip Bench				
Skull Crushers				

Notes:

_____

_____

_____

_____

_____

_____

_____

Week - 8	Day Date	Max Inc Bar	Number of Sets	How I Feel
Squat				
Standing Press				
Bent Over Rows				
Bench Press				
Inclined Press				
Standing Bicep Curl				
Reverse Curl				
Close Grip Bench				
Skull Crushers				

Notes:

_____

_____

_____

_____

_____

_____

_____

Week - 9	Day Date	Max Inc Bar	Number of Sets	How I Feel
Squat				

Standing Press				

Bent Over Rows				

Bench Press				
Inclined Press				

Standing Bicep Curl				
Reverse Curl				

Close Grip Bench				
Skull Crushers				

Notes:

_____

_____

_____

_____

_____

_____

_____

Week - 10	Day Date	Max Inc Bar	Number of Sets	How I Feel
Squat				
Standing Press				
Bent Over Rows				
Bench Press Inclined Press				
Standing Bicep Curl Reverse Curl				
Close Grip Bench Skull Crushers				

Notes:

_____

_____

_____

_____

_____

_____

_____

Week - 11	Day Date	Max Inc Bar	Number of Sets	How I Feel
Squat				

Standing Press				

Bent Over Rows				

Bench Press				
Inclined Press				

Standing Bicep Curl				
Reverse Curl				

Close Grip Bench				
Skull Crushers				

Notes:

_____

_____

_____

_____

_____

_____

_____

Week - 12	Day Date	Max Inc Bar	Number of Sets	How I Feel
Squat				

Standing Press				

Bent Over Rows				

Bench Press				
Inclined Press				

Standing Bicep Curl				
Reverse Curl				

Close Grip Bench				
Skull Crushers				

Notes:

_____

_____

_____

_____

_____

_____

_____

Week - 13	Day	Max	Number	How I
	Date	Inc Bar	of Sets	Feel
Squat				

Standing Press				

Bent Over Rows				

Bench Press				
Inclined Press				

Standing Bicep Curl				
Reverse Curl				

Close Grip Bench				
Skull Crushers				

Notes:

_____

_____

_____

_____

_____

_____

_____

Week - 14	Day Date	Max Inc Bar	Number of Sets	How I Feel
Squat				
Standing Press				
Bent Over Rows				
Bench Press				
Inclined Press				
Standing Bicep Curl				
Reverse Curl				
Close Grip Bench				
Skull Crushers				

Notes:

_____

_____

_____

_____

_____

_____

_____

Week - 15	Day Date	Max Inc Bar	Number of Sets	How I Feel
Squat				

Standing Press				

Bent Over Rows				

Bench Press				
Inclined Press				

Standing Bicep Curl				
Reverse Curl				

Close Grip Bench				
Skull Crushers				

Notes:

_____

_____

_____

_____

_____

_____

_____

Week - 16	Day Date	Max Inc Bar	Number of Sets	How I Feel
Squat				
Standing Press				
Bent Over Rows				
Bench Press Inclined Press				
Standing Bicep Curl Reverse Curl				
Close Grip Bench Skull Crushers				

Notes:

_____

_____

_____

_____

_____

_____

_____

Week - 17	Day Date	Max Inc Bar	Number of Sets	How I Feel
Squat				
Standing Press				
Bent Over Rows				
Bench Press				
Inclined Press				
Standing Bicep Curl				
Reverse Curl				
Close Grip Bench				
Skull Crushers				

Notes:

_____

_____

_____

_____

_____

_____

_____

Week - 18	Day Date	Max Inc Bar	Number of Sets	How I Feel
Squat				

	Day Date	Max Inc Bar	Number of Sets	How I Feel
Standing Press				

	Day Date	Max Inc Bar	Number of Sets	How I Feel
Bent Over Rows				

	Day Date	Max Inc Bar	Number of Sets	How I Feel
Bench Press				
Inclined Press				

	Day Date	Max Inc Bar	Number of Sets	How I Feel
Standing Bicep Curl				
Reverse Curl				

	Day Date	Max Inc Bar	Number of Sets	How I Feel
Close Grip Bench				
Skull Crushers				

Notes:

_____

_____

_____

_____

_____

_____

_____

Week - 19	Day Date	Max Inc Bar	Number of Sets	How I Feel
Squat				
Standing Press				
Bent Over Rows				
Bench Press				
Inclined Press				
Standing Bicep Curl				
Reverse Curl				
Close Grip Bench				
Skull Crushers				

Notes:

_____

_____

_____

_____

_____

_____

_____

Week - 20	Day Date	Max Inc Bar	Number of Sets	How I Feel
Squat				
Standing Press				
Bent Over Rows				
Bench Press				
Inclined Press				
Standing Bicep Curl				
Reverse Curl				
Close Grip Bench				
Skull Crushers				

Notes:

_____

_____

_____

_____

_____

_____

_____

Week - 21	Day Date	Max Inc Bar	Number of Sets	How I Feel
Squat				
Standing Press				
Bent Over Rows				
Bench Press				
Inclined Press				
Standing Bicep Curl				
Reverse Curl				
Close Grip Bench				
Skull Crushers				

Notes:

_____

_____

_____

_____

_____

_____

_____

| Week - 22 | Day | Max | Number | How I |

	Date	Inc Bar	of Sets	Feel
Squat				

Standing Press				

Bent Over Rows				

Bench Press				
Inclined Press				

Standing Bicep Curl				
Reverse Curl				

Close Grip Bench				
Skull Crushers				

Notes:

_____

_____

_____

_____

_____

_____

_____

Week - 23	Day Date	Max Inc Bar	Number of Sets	How I Feel
Squat				

Standing Press				

Bent Over Rows				

Bench Press				
Inclined Press				

Standing Bicep Curl				
Reverse Curl				

Close Grip Bench				
Skull Crushers				

Notes:

_____

_____

_____

_____

_____

_____

_____

Week - 24	Day Date	Max Inc Bar	Number of Sets	How I Feel
Squat				
Standing Press				
Bent Over Rows				
Bench Press Inclined Press				
Standing Bicep Curl Reverse Curl				
Close Grip Bench Skull Crushers				

Notes:

_____

_____

_____

_____

_____

_____

_____

Week - 25	Day Date	Max Inc Bar	Number of Sets	How I Feel
Squat				

Standing Press				

Bent Over Rows				

Bench Press				
Inclined Press				

Standing Bicep Curl				
Reverse Curl				

Close Grip Bench				
Skull Crushers				

Notes:

_____

_____

_____

_____

_____

_____

_____

Week - 26	Day Date	Max Inc Bar	Number of Sets	How I Feel
Squat				
Standing Press				
Bent Over Rows				
Bench Press Inclined Press				
Standing Bicep Curl Reverse Curl				
Close Grip Bench Skull Crushers				

Notes:

_____

_____

_____

_____

_____

_____

_____

www.ingramcontent.com/pod-product-compliance
Lightning Source LLC
Chambersburg PA
CBHW070337290526
45791CB00003B/1363